Diabolically Delicious

Our Toxic Relationship with Food

Angela Johnson

Contents

Preface

November 21, 2016

My Dearest Love,

I guess it's not appropriate to ask "How are you?" You're always fine and doing what you do, nothing ever affects you. I'm just checking in to share with you how I'm doing, not that you really care. You probably see where this is going.

So here it is my love, my best friend, you and I go way back. As a matter of fact, my very first experience with you was in my mother's womb. I needed you to survive even then! You know me better than I know myself. You are always there to supply what I'm missing. You are there for me whatever the emotion, situation or event. I can always count on you when no one else is or has been there for me. You don't need any explanation and you definitely don't do the judgment thing. You go straight to the emotion because you know me so well. You always know just where it hurts. I have come to depend on you for everything.

We have had so many amazing moments together, just us. Oh my goodness, your versatility is priceless, I can never get bored with you, you take care of that too. You just seem to make everything better, every single time. I mean you are perfect and ever evolving. You have this amazing ability to comfort me and satisfy almost every craving. Just when I think I've had enough of you, you come up with a different variation of yourself. You get the job done every single time and won't stop until you have satisfied me completely. You, my love, are an amazing force that I felt I was no match for. You have rendered me powerless. I mean, simply stated you're right there with God! Ok, who am I fooling? YOU ARE GOD!! Wait, did I just say that?! Really?! Ok so let me regroup as I wipe the tears from my eyes, this just got real!

You, my love, seemed to know everything about me, while I hardly knew anything about you. Being honest, as I look back at my life, how is it possible that you are always available no matter the time, day, hour, situation, whenever, it doesn't matter, you're there! You gave me exactly what I needed at that time. I mean who can do that, who can be that? Who can be that tuned in to my very being?! YOU! Yes, you were my God, my EVERYTHING!! I put you before I put Him. Everything that God is, is what you were to me. Once I came to that realization, I had to repent and ask God for His forgiveness. You were truly my idol. I actually even knew you better than I knew God.

I couldn't give you a bible verse, but I could tell you exactly where you were at any given time. I couldn't tell you God's promises, but I knew that 9 times out of 10 you delivered what you promised. You're so easy to find and always where I want you and when I want you. You make me feel how I need to feel, when I need to feel it. You make me take a deep breath, exhale and relax in your goodness. You actually have the ability to make the noise stop, the hurt and the pain to go away. You always allow me to escape in you. You don't judge me, cuss me out, debate with me, laugh at me, nor argue with me. You usually give me your undivided attention unless someone interrupts us and wants to find out what we've got going on. You soothe me, listen to me, and are there for me tangibly without fail. I can always put my hands on you, every single time as far back as I can remember. How can I not be in love with something or someone like that? You are everything, and I simply cannot live without you in my life or I will die. I am truly addicted to you, and I need help. The time has come where it is seriously time that I re-evaluate this toxic relationship that I have somehow confused with love, nourishment, fulfilment, and caring.

My dearest Food, I've come to realize that you were just a bit too perfect. By me becoming so dependent upon you, I was letting myself go and dishonoring God. What happened? How did I get here? Why was I chunky? Why didn't I want to participate in life? Why, when I looked around me, my body was different than other girls my age? Why couldn't I wear the same size clothes as my mom? Why was I younger than her, but weighed more than she did? Why was I getting teased and bullied when I was at school when I would eat my lunch? Why didn't my PE uniform fit like everyone else's did? Why was my mom always trying to restrict my food consumption, all while bringing in unhealthy food, only to tell me I couldn't have any? Why did I have to shop in a different clothing section for plus size teens? Why was I always sneaking and having you to myself, when no one was watching.

Situation: When I was about 11 or 12, I had daily/weekly chores that I had to perform when I came home from school. Now my mom was a rather thin shapely size 4 – 6. She never struggled with her

weight or food addiction of any kind, however, she could put it away but never gained weight. So when she wanted her treats, she had no problem buying them and they would last for months at a time. Not on my watch! So she would buy certain items that would be off limits to me, because she knew I loved to eat. I thought it was cruel and unusual punishment to bring food in the house only to tell me I couldn't have any. Not cool! So one day my task was to defrost the freezer old school style, where you empty it out and place a boiling hot pot of water in the freezer to melt the ice. Well there was ice cream in the freezer that had been in there too long for my liking. So when it came time to defrost the freezer, I decided I was going to eradicate that ice cream (which by the way is my number one vice) that had been tempting me for way too long. When my mom came home she asked me what happened to the ice cream. I lied and told her that it had molded and I had to throw it away. She

never made a comment about it. It was years later as a process of my healing that it came out that I actually ate the ice cream, because clearly ice cream doesn't mold. It may get frost bitten, but it wasn't even that. Clearly, she knew I had a problem.

Through it all you never made fun of me, you just comforted me and were there for me at all times. As I got older and began to understand that whatever happened, you were there for me. You were only a temporary comfort that lasted only for the moment. Then when you did what you were there to do, I was left with some sort of shame and guilt, discomfort in my body, emotionally lonely and insecure. Somehow, you would make your way right back in and the cycle would start all over again.

Situation: I was clearing out the fridge and freezer of all food that didn't serve me well. Hubby and I got into a heated conversation and I got totally stressed out. After he left the kitchen I went in the

trash can and got out a chocolate dessert that I had thrown away! *Wednesday.Thursday.Friday!!....***Is that crazy or what? And let me tell you when I took that first bite, everything within me just relaxed. I exhaled and it was like a drug and I had just had a fix. Then I was able to carry on with the rest of my day.**

In seeking help, I began to realize that I was in a F.O.G (Food Over God) placing you above God. I had to go to someone who had more power than you. I had to go to your creator. I had to do a background check. I had to find out who I was really in a relationship with and why I was so controlled by you. How are you omniscient and omnipresent in my life? Something that I was always taught was only for God. Something was desperately wrong, I literally felt like my life was out of control and I was just grasping for breath and some type of solace from this toxic relationship.

This is what you didn't know. Remember when I told you I needed to be free of you and the power and control you had over my life? In desperation, I went to OUR CREATOR, who turned out to be the one and only GOD! I asked Him to deliver me from this unhealthy, ungodly relationship I had with you. He began to slowly and ever so beautifully show me how I had put so much trust in you and not in Him, especially when it came to my emotions. He began to answer my call for help by showing me how to first understand the order of things. That if I wanted to be delivered/free of my addiction from you, I had to first put all of my trust and faith in Him because He created you, and knows you better than you know yourself. Therefore, if I wanted to find out how to be delivered/free from you, I had to find out all about you and understand the control you had over my life.

I began to pray and ask the Lord to show me who you really were, and He did just that. He showed me how you did what you did. He showed me who your parents were, come to find out they were Sugar and Flour, last name Satan. He showed me how much power and influence they had over your life. He showed me your siblings, and cousins, such as Processed, GMO's, Iodized Salt, Grains, Fake Dairy and Artificial Ingredients. Granted some of your relatives are not as diabolical as you are, but some of them can be turned up too!

I began to see the crazy, truly dysfunctional type of life you really came from, and how crazy and dysfunctional I had become because of you, but you still had this amazing ability to mask yourself in almost everything you did, because you seemed so perfect at all times. You've always known that I needed you to survive, but because ultimately you have no feelings or emotional attachment to me, it was easy for you to play this cruel trick on my life. So as the Lord began to show me who you really were, I let Him know that I still needed you to survive so what was I supposed to do.

What was the plan for me now? The healing process continued with trust, guidance, and listening to His voice for direction, He began to place people and resources in my life that could help me as well. He then introduced me to some long lost, not so popular relatives of yours who are kind of like the black sheep of the family. Nobody really fancies them because they don't have the swag and charm as the Satan Family. They are called the Healthy's. Fruit and Veggie, last name Healthy. Their offspring were too many to name, but here are a few....Whole, Natural, Unprocessed, Asparagus, Broccoli, Tomato, Avocado, Sweet Potato, Cucumber, Apple, Orange, Water, Pineapple, Nuts, Eggs, Real Dairy and the list goes on. He also introduced me to their friends the Exercise family.

Ultimately, I've decided that our toxic relationship has come to an end. I no longer depend on you for my source of comfort, I have God for that now. Being that I know what you're really made of and how I have allowed you to affect my life in such an unhealthy way, I began to associate myself with the Healthy Family and the Exercise Family, and they are not detrimental to my well- being. They are more balanced and know their place in my life. They are not aggressive nor boisterous in our relationship. They bring me peace, clarity, balance and stability. They don't wear out their welcome, and are quite respectful and nourishing, gentle and loving to my very being. We have established boundaries that we are both comfortable with. They honor OUR CREATOR, and don't ever overstep their position in my life. It's a beautiful fit, and a much healthier and functional relationship.

The fact of the matter is this; you will always be a part of my life, but by the grace of God, I have been able to place realistic boundaries on your involvement in my life. I know exactly who you are and what you are capable of and I know you will never change. As a matter of fact, you just keep getting progressively worse, so I keep my distance. I could never hate you, it's just that

my relationship with you as I knew it, is
OVER.

Warmly,
Angie

Introduction

You may want to go back and read at least the first half of that letter again to realize that I am seriously talking about food.

Are you ready to face the reality that most of the food we are consuming is diabolically delicious and that you honestly have a toxic relationship with food? Are you ready to be healed?

Are you at that point?

I mean face it, food is a part of our everyday life, we absolutely can't live without it, let's not kid ourselves. Every event that we go to, almost every situation that we're in, it has an impact on us. So think about some of the events we've been through in our lives. If your relationship goes bad, if we have an argument with someone, if we have a bad day at work, if life throws us curve balls that we don't have the capacity to handle, we get depressed, we get happy, we get adventurous, we get nervous, and the list goes on and on……what do we turn to? Often, it's food. I know RIGHT?!?!?! Next thing we know, we've gained a bunch of weight, our clothes fit differently, we have zero energy, zero patience, zero tolerance, our sleep patterns are off, our bodies are sore and stiff, our emotions are out of control, and the situation that we are going through or experiencing is still there. Per adventure it's a person that we're having problems with in the relationship, they are not liking us so much and we're liking ourselves even less than that! The relationship gets worse. And yet again we turn to the very thing that seems to never fail us even more so……FOOD!! It's a vicious cycle that starts all over again.

If we're totally honest and transparent with ourselves, I think we all know, deep down inside of us, this is not how we should be living, this is not how we want to function in this life. Seriously, food is everywhere, and if you're like I was, food may very well be considered your best friend! You also may have developed that toxic relationship with the food. I want to be here for you today to tell you, that this doesn't have to be anymore. You see, I'm so delighted to be in the place that I am now, rather than where I started out.

Growing up an only child, I was kind of the loner in my family. My experience as an only child was a rather lonely existence. I pretty much felt invisible, I didn't talk much, didn't have many friends, nor did I have a healthy relationship with my parents. There was a lot of silence and solitude in my life. I learned early on that food came through for me every time. It was pretty much the only thing I had in my life that I got some type of solace from. It never disappointed. The problem was that I just could never get enough of it. What I came to find out is that it wasn't the "food" per se, that I was so enamored with, but the way it made me "feel". It took the pain away, even when I wasn't aware that I was in pain. Before I knew it, every time something went down, or an emotion that I was experiencing made me feel some type of way, I would be coupled up with my best friend! By the way, I must mention that I didn't even have a "real" best friend, so this was a real thing for me. From my understanding, a best friend is non-judgmental, but will set you straight when needed, you can share anything with them, you laugh with them, they have a way of making you feel better, and always there in the time of need, they love you no matter what, true blue, through and through!

 Fast forward and now I'm 18 and still rather chunky by my and societal standards. I think I was basing my body size off of what my mom's body size was, which was a cool size 6, to my not so cool size 12-14! At this point I'm a senior in high school, some kind of way I turned out to be pretty popular. However, I still considered myself to be "fat", (If I knew then what I know now, I would love to be "fat" again!) I weighed 170 pounds and was 5ft 7in tall. Keep in mind this was in the 80's when size 0 – 4 was the "in" size and anything beyond that was by the female standard considered fat, but the guys considered me "thick". You know how we are as women, so insecure about how we look and it's most often based on our female peers that we seek approval from. If we don't look like "Slim Sally" over there, then we are not the right size. If we're honest with ourselves, not much has changed with us, because we are still basing our beauty standards on the standards of other women in society. And now this diabolical thing called "social media" has us all twisted up, confused and acting all crazy, trying to look like the celebrities and those fake photos on IG and FB, and whatever else they are creating to keep us never being satisfied with the natural beauty of who we really are.

Please understand that we are making wise decisions based on lies ladies! What do I mean by that?? Go with me down this road for a moment, if you will. Right now, yes right now, pick up your phone that's right next to you, go to an Instagram picture of someone that you may look at and say, "Hey, she's flawless, look at her skin, look at how beautiful her face is. Oh my God that body on her, how is that possible? She must eat perfectly and work out 24/7. Her breasts are perfect, her curves are in all the right places, Oh….My….God…..look at her…. butt! So unfair!! I so wish I could look like that." Now what does that make you want to do, how does that make you feel? (it makes ME say EF it cuz I will never look like that and go out and "treat" myself to a bomb ass greasy, juicy cheeseburger, fries (extra crispy) and the most decadent shake they make, but that's just me) It could actually be several things by the time I'm done. I'm sorry I digress, I had a moment, now let's take a look at the mass amounts of makeup on these women. Look at the bodies that they are showing off. Most of the time none of this is real!! PLEASE UNDERSTAND!! Make up: they are wearing a ton of it, and you see the layers that they are crazy enough to spend hours applying and you watching the whole process, but yet and still we want to look like them. In my opinion some of this stuff is sheer witchcraft, oh my God and the men that are fooled by them! Hair: really, who has time to spend on hair looking like this without a hair out of place, full of body and perfectly healthy? You want that style, you go to your stylist and say, I want this style, make it happen. They in turn look at you like you're crazy and say, "You know that's a weave, right?" Ok whatever, still, make it happen! Seriously?!?!. Body: perfect measurements, everything in proportion. Breasts: sheer perfection, perfect in size and shape, oh yeah and no bra really?!?! Knock it off, how'd you do that without paying for them babies (especially after having some babies)? Don't get me wrong, beautiful breasts are magical, knock yourself out, if I could, I would probably buy me some too, or at least perk up the ones I already have! Now keep in mind the angle of the camera. That is EVERYTHING!! Seriously, how many selfies do we take, and how many countless angles do we try before we post even ONE selfie?!? Ok so then, you have this amazing discovery called "Photoshop" the most fabulous invention ever, how do they come up with this stuff?! They have photoshop apps now that work off of your original picture, and by the time they're done with all of those filters and editing the pic, they don't even remotely look like themselves, yet we want to look like them. NOTHING IS REAL!! Please understand that. Stop basing your standard of beauty on someone else's fakeness. It's all a mirage, be you and be ok with that. YOU ARE BEAUTIFUL NATURALLY. Now don't get me wrong some of us need more help than others and that's ok. Just take care of yourself from the inside out and you will be amazed at how beautiful you truly are NATURALLY.

Ok so I just had to give you a quick reality check. Now by this time I've met my amazing husband, well he wasn't so amazing at the time, he was just a cool dude that paid attention to me, now he's exceeded AMAZING. We had a lot of growing to do.

So ultimately, we begin dating and loving on each other, just having loads of fun as new couples tend to do. What is ALWAYS involved in the dating process? That's right…….FOOD! And for some reason, it's as if food has never tasted so good. You are trying all of the restaurants you were too cheap to check out on your own. Then you begin to experiment with different tastes and venues, you start going out of town and eating all over the place! Next thing you know those pants you used to wear when you first started dating, are rather snug. That waistline and booty starts spreading out a bit more. You are more comfortable in the relationship at this point so your outfits begin to change and be a little less tight. As a matter of fact, they downright don't fit any more PERIOD! You already know when he picks you up, you are going to get something to eat, and it's going to be diabolically delicious, even if it's a burger, simply because you are with him. So you tell yourself, "stop playing, I'm gonna make sure I'm wearing something comfy and stretchy, because we are about to throw down!"

Adulting

The ebbs and flows of my life began to happen. I graduated from High School, college was an unfulfilled desire and in less than a year I was married. I began having children and one thing just led to another and my body just kept expanding. All the while, even though I was very active with my family, friends, work and church (which is where I gained a substantial amount of weight because I got super comfortable) I just couldn't get a grip on my eating. By this time I had probably tried 80% of the diets that were known to be "effective." I took HCG shots, I got my teeth wired, I did the cabbage soup diet, the boiled egg diet, the cookie diet, Atkins, South Beach, Nutrisystem, Weight Watchers, you name it, I no doubt tried it. I counted calories, took pills, I even took pills that promised you could eat WHATEVER you wanted and still lose poundage. Guess what???.......it worked until it didn't anymore, but I was still trying to eat whatever I wanted, but I obviously didn't get the memo when they changed the formula of the product. So mean. At some point in this craziness, I found out I had gallstones. I don't wish that pain on anyone. I eventually changed my diet because of it. The "plus side" (pun intended) to that, is that I lost a lot of weight, because at that point almost anything I ate made me sick. After my 3rd child was born, I got my gallbladder removed. The fact of the matter is that I couldn't wait to be able to eat the foods that I was restricted from for so long. And because of that I gained all of the weight that I had lost and some. Why and how??? Because through all of that, I never changed my mindset about food. There were several times that I wished I had never gotten it removed, stayed sick and just dealt with the pain of it all, but at least I would've kept the weight off.

Then I began to realize food had me so out of control of my life that something drastically had to change. I was depressed all the time and just felt like I was never happy and tired all of the time. Exhausted from always trying to lose weight, exercise, drink water etc., and nothing I did was working. I prayed to God that He would deliver me from this emotional rollercoaster of eating that I was continually on and He did just that!

The Transformation

Most of us are familiar with the occurrence of Adam and Eve, at least the food part. We all know that when Adam and Eve ate of the fruit of the tree that was forbidden in the garden,(which by the way I think were figs and not an apple, because when they realized they were naked, they covered themselves with fig leaves) that's when all hell broke loose and we've been doomed ever since, especially when it comes to food and our relationship with it. By the way, the tragedy was not in full effect until Adam ate of the fruit. Eve partook first but nothing was put in effect at that time, not until she gave it to Adam and he did eat.(Gen.3:6-7) From this account, you can see how food has played an integral part of our very being, all the way since the beginning of time and it has affected how we function with it ever since. God said, "the day you eat of the fruit from the tree of the knowledge of good and evil, you shall surely die". Think for a moment, if you will, we have been dying from it ever since. Primarily because of the way we abuse it and don't know how to establish healthy boundaries with it. Also because of all of the chemicals that are currently in the food that we consume. A lot of it is cloaked behind healthy and nutritious and it couldn't be farther from the truth. Especially when you factor in all of the food related diseases and illnesses that we are experiencing in this day and time. The way the food companies process food, it is designed to continually make us crave it and want more of it, this of course making them wealthier. So be assured that you are not crazy when you have these insane cravings for things and you don't understand why. It's really chemical and hormonal. Even in biblical days, people died over food for various reasons and not because it was processed in a lab.

Prayer Answered!

Enter the beginning of my life changing journey. I was walking one day, which is usually the time that I pray and set my intentions for the day or the week. I was telling the Lord that I was simply exhausted, that this is not my body that I am living in and that my purpose was to be a voice and a help and or support for overweight women who felt they had no voice, help or support, but who would listen to me when I was so fat and out of shape. I asked Him to please help me and change my mind on how I thought about food, please change my toxic relationship that I had with food. Help me to not depend on it for everything, help me to trust Him for my solace and solution to this never ending dilemma. Out of nowhere this woman walks up to me and begins talking to me. In my mind, I was like look lady, I'm minding my own business, not bothering anyone, I'm having a moment so leave me alone! I didn't say all of that, but that is what I was thinking. So, as I decided to take my guards down and listen to her, the first thing she did when she approached me was said hello and show me a brochure of a 12- step program, that read, "are you a food addict?" Immediately I was offended, and was thinking like, hey lady, are you saying I'm fat? Then within seconds I realized this could be an answer to my prayers, and quickly "let go of my ego". I was like "Lord that was super-fast!" As we began to walk together, she began to share with me how the program worked. By this time, we had walked to her house and she began to show me pictures at her previous size, and I was floored! I asked how do I get signed up and when can I start? She gave me all of the pertinent information and I was at the meeting that same night! I was so excited, and felt like there was hope for me after all and that God had truly heard my cry and answered my prayers.

The program was named FA. Food Addicts in Recovery Anonymous. (foodaddicts.org) Life changing for me! Exactly what I needed to get my life together. I think one of the things that really made it worth trying was that it was FREE!! What?!?!? It gets no better!! I had spent thousands of dollars on diets and weight loss products, I even got the Lap Band procedure done and that didn't even work! Where I heard screeching brakes was when she told me that they abstain COMPLETELY from all sugar and flour, wait it gets better. Also, they weighed and measured every meal, no snacks in between, *W*ednesday.*T*hursday.*F*riday?!?!? Then she proceeded to give me a list of all that the program entailed of, and yes, I was overwhelmed! At that point, I was ready to run for the hills, and yes run away from yet another "diet plan". The fact of the matter was that it really was not a diet plan at all, it was a lifestyle, which is completely different. A diet is temporary, a lifestyle is something that you should be able to do for the rest and or the majority of your life. So I jumped right in, it was one of the most difficult things I had ever done in my life, but by far the most courageous, rewarding, fulfilling, and successful. I successfully stayed on track for 4 months. Let me tell you, I made it through my birthday, Halloween, Thanksgiving, Christmas, New Year and Valentine's Day! I lost around 50lbs effortlessly and was the happiest I had ever been. Yes, I had my typical struggles because as we all know that when you are addicted to something, there is a detox period that you go through when you are desiring to come clean. There was so much that the program required of me, mentally and spiritually, but I managed to pull it off until I couldn't anymore. Also I, along with my husband are the owners of a very successful breakfast and soul food restaurant. So mind you, I was operating like an alcoholic that worked at a bar! When I tell you the mere stress of that business combined with the amazing food that we have, in the beginning most days I had a really hard time, but the tools that I learned in FA helped me to stay on track at some of my weakest moments. Imagine my day to day struggles. Nonetheless, I had an amazing sponsor and I kept on going and I managed my life the best way I knew how, I didn't deviate what so ever, I made my adjustments and stayed on program.

What I realized is that with all the crazy that was going on in my life, the only thing that I had COMPLETE control over, was what I chose to put in my mouth! That was one of the most liberating feelings I had personally felt. I mean, I couldn't control my husband, my children, my employees, I couldn't control the weather, the events of the world, and I definitely couldn't control what people thought of me. So when I realized the only thing I could truly control was what I put in my mouth, it was so incredibly satisfying and empowering. From that, I was able to control my emotions, and the way I ate and the way I thought about food, I was able to control the relationship that I had with food. I learned so much about how food becomes so toxic to our very being, from the way it is prepared to our relationship with it. It was no longer a "frenemy" but something that I was able to manage and not be afraid of. Being in this program was truly the start of my healthy relationship with food. It was truly food freedom. I had to begin to "deal" with my issues, current and times past. I had to learn how to "not eat over" my issues and face them head on. Was it a painful process? Most definitely, but the growth and the life changes that I experienced were priceless. I learned so much about who I was as a person and what I was capable of accomplishing. I no longer ran away from life and became an active participant. So much positivity entered my life. My total vibration changed regarding what I was inviting into my life. I slept like a baby, I was so much more patient with EVERYTHING and EVERYONE I encountered. I took up Yoga, Pilates, Zumba, I began to take various dance classes, swim, walk, hike and bike ride. Oh my goodness, and let me not forget to mention that I was beginning to buy clothing of a smaller size! That part right there was one of the biggest rewards of all. I was able to cross my legs, my thighs were not rubbing profusely! It was truly an amazing experience. My back stopped hurting, my knees were not tight and hurting, my ankles were not swollen, all of the inflammation had left my body and all was well with the world during that phase of my life.

The Journey Continues

There comes a time in everyone's life where at some point you get off track. You look at where you are, then think about where you were, especially if it was a good place, then you look back and say, "What the hell happened? How did I get back here again?"

So……….. when I did that amazing 12-step program that I absolutely swear by, (I still do to this day) I lost focus and began to overwhelm myself with the rigidity of it. I felt like I could no longer participate in all of the restrictions that the program entailed of. I began to lie to my sponsor, and with that became this incredible guilt. I'm not a liar and it was going against my very core. It wasn't that I was re-establishing a toxic relationship, and going back to my old habits, because I had learned to create these incredible boundaries, and had learned how to eat properly and read labels, etc., but I just began to go off "program" and that was not in line with the program guidelines.

I began to have this extra taste of a different type of freedom which entailed of not having to report to anyone, not having to have designated times for meals, not having to pack my food for long days, or unexpected situations where I didn't know what I would be faced with when it came down to meal time. I didn't have to weigh and measure all of my food anymore, I could take random spur of the moment trips with my friends and family. I felt this new sense of liberation, in my newly developing thinner frame. I could add things that I couldn't have on the program, within moderation of course. Did I say moderation? Everybody knows you can't tell an addict to "use" in moderation something they are addicted to.

UH OH......so at this point we have now established a failure to communicate! Do you tell an alcoholic to drink in moderation, or a sugar addict to have sugar in moderation, or a food addict to eat in moderation? I think NOT! However, in most cases with the exception of all other addictions, yes we do! Slowly but surely I totally began to eliminate most of the practices that I learned and that worked so very well for me, and started slipping back into my old way of thinking and eating. Well let's elaborate on that a little more. Don't let the smooth taste fool you. Food is so smooth and fun, you really don't see the damage that we allow it to cause. Food is harmless, I mean we totally need it to survive, we absolutely cannot live without it. We would surely die if we didn't have it. We don't think about being addicted to sugar, or just food in general. We don't want to face the reality that that might really be a thing! After all, food is the only addiction on the planet that we cannot live without. If you list all of the addictions that are in existence, and there are countless, it would actually stun you, but food is the ONLY one that you can't survive without. Let's face it, we can't live without air or water, true enough, but we won't go as far as to say we are addicted to it.

Often, food becomes our solace, that friend that we turn to when we are stressed or sad, or having any kind of struggle. There are transitions in life. At every transition, I get the opportunity to find out who I am. What are the things that I like? What are the things that I dislike? It teaches me how to take better care of myself. I'm finally at a place in my life where I'm learning to get comfortable in my own skin. The ways that I have done that is through various soul searching processes. Some fun, some not so fun. I take mini "soul sabbaticals" (mini trips, alone or with my husband) When he's the source of my stress, that's when I go alone! I listen to music that absolutely nourishes my spirit, I dance alone, in the mirror and just have fun with it! I take walks and listen to my books on my phone. I take detox baths, I get massages, I take cooking classes, I teach cooking classes, I read loads of self-help books, (that's the part that can be not so fun) I conduct movement classes for women who are overweight and it's difficult for them to move around in their bodies. Find what works for you and begin to do that, your mind, body and soul will thank you for it. We have been blessed to have this body, it's the only one we have, and we are fearfully and wonderfully made and we should treat our bodies with the love and respect that it so deserves. We don't even realize how hard our bodies work for us every single day, just to simply breathe. Then when we add all of the additional weight to it, and the lack of nourishment that we supply it with, it's a wonder that it just doesn't give up on us, and sometimes it does! If you look around you today, that is exactly what it is doing, giving up on us because we've given up on it. It is so gracious to us. Imagine if we had to carry around 100 extra pounds in our arms or on our backs every single day! How long do you think we could physically do that? Like I couldn't even lift 100lbs, let alone carry it around daily. Think about when and if you've ever been to the gym and they have all of those dumbbells, lying around. Have you ever just picked up a 50lb weight? I bet you couldn't pick up another one in the other hand and walk around with it, at least not for long. I challenge you to try it the next time you come across some weights. See how much weight you can physically pick up and carry. Then think of how much extra weight you are carrying on your body and then thank God for His goodness and mercy!

Ultimately, I have learned to do what serves me and my well-being. I place myself in positive environments with positive people. The moment I don't feel right about the company I am around, or the environment that I'm in, when the opportunity presents itself, I dismiss myself, or don't participate in the first place. Why??? Because I can, and so can YOU!

Situation: Hubby and I had gone up the coast in our convertible and had just had an amazing lunch on the beach, on the way back, as fate would have it some kind of way it went south. He had pissed me off about something and of course he was

in chill mode, because clearly it was my issue and not his. So instead of going the rest of the way home feeling uneasy and not in a positive energy field, I decided that I didn't have to ride the rest of the way home with him. So he happened to stop off and make a purchase somewhere. He went inside the store and I exited the vehicle. I called an Uber and went home. He came back to the car only to realize I was not in it. He called to check on me, and I told him I took Uber home. He said "ok, just checking on you, get home safely." Typically I would've gone home and ate profusely because I was upset, but instead, I made my adjustments early on and did not have the desire to replace my emotions with food. That's called a non-scale victory!

Now, you would think that because of all that I've learned and all I've shared so far, that I live an easy life when it comes to food but as I stated previously, I'm a restaurant owner. So every day I have to fight the urge to indulge. I'm learning how to be conscious and aware of my food choices. What does it really mean to eat healthy? In a nutshell, try your best to eliminate as much processed food as you possibly can. Which pretty much means anything in a package, and that has more than 5 ingredients, and especially ones you can't even pronounce! I've learned a lot and I'm so excited to live as a much healthier individual than I used to. I'm still overweight, but I'm much healthier and I'm moving in the right direction.

Some of the things that I have found to be helpful are as follows:

- Meal prepping (this is a really big deal)

- Meal planning for the week

- Cooking your own meals at home

- Not eating out as often as you typically would

- When you do dine out, take a look at the online menu of the establishment you are about to visit and see what offerings they have, that you would feel comfortable with. And if you're not comfortable, depending on the occasion, maybe suggest another restaurant to attend. Also know that it's ok to say no when invited to dine out. Take control of your own actions. No one can make you go eat somewhere that does not fit what you are doing. If you go, it's your choice, so dine responsibly.

- Respectfully and kindly ask your server lots of questions regarding the way certain foods are prepared. It also helps to let them know up front that you are sensitive to the way food is prepared and that you will be asking them several questions. That way they don't get too annoyed. Sometimes they know and sometimes they don't, so when in doubt leave it out!

- If you are really craving a certain item that you have not had in a very long time, and you just can't shake the craving. Depending on where you are in your journey, go OUT and get that item. Consume it there, and do not bring any of it back into your home. Whatever is not consumed there, step away from the item and be done with it. Whatever you do, DO NOT BRING IT BACK HOME WITH YOU. So make sure you only get enough for a single serving. If it is something that is not a single serving, you have a few options. A) don't get it. B) eat what you want and throw the rest away (this is not the time to be thinking of all of the starving people in the world). C) make sure you go with a friend that you can share with. D) simply ask the server to remove the item from your table

- When dining out, ask for a take-out container as soon as your food arrives so that you can make a second or third meal out of it.

- Split a meal with your dining partner, that's given you both want to try the same thing.

- Ask for a smaller plate and take some of the food from your entrée and place it on the smaller plate.

- Don't allow them to bring the bread basket. Sometimes it's easier to resist when it never makes it to the table in the first place.

- If you're dining out and all else fails and you can't pull the plug, have a stop loss plan in action. Tell someone that you're with to help you out by pouring salt or water all over the food. I typically don't have enough power to do this on my own, so I will tell someone I'm with to do it for me, when I have made known to them that I am having a moment and I need to be reeled back in. People are usually pretty eager to help you and they take pleasure in pouring salt or water in your plate for the sake of helping you out. Or they will simply take it home with them. They wanted what you ordered anyway!

Situation: One day I wanted some ice cream really bad, and ice cream is my kryptonite! So I couldn't shake the craving, and I was not going to be able to rest until I had some. I went to the kitchen, got me a spoon, left the house, went to the grocery store and purchased a half gallon of ONE of my favorite flavors. I drove to the park that I frequent when I "exercise", sat right in front of it and had my ice cream. I didn't get a pint because I knew I would be looking for more when that was gone, so I didn't even play with

it. I almost finished the half gallon, then that moment of choice came for me to either sit there and finish it until I got sick, take the rest of it home with me because it was just too good to throw away, or yes throw it away and live to see another day without ice cream in the house. So I did the responsible thing and threw it away. Yes I littered and left the mess for someone else to clean up instead of me! It felt pretty darn good I must say. I would call that a non-scale victory! Even though I may have just consumed 1000+ calories!

I haven't always made these choices and it hasn't always been that way, nor easy. As you can imagine from my letter, I've had some issues with food. At my lowest point, honestly, it felt like I was eating 24/7. I was obsessed with food; it was all I could think about. The only shows I wanted to watch on TV were the food/cooking shows. I even started keeping a log of places that I wanted to visit in different parts of the world for when we traveled. Where could I go today? What drive-thru could I have for breakfast, lunch or dinner? I kept snacks on me, my car, my purse, my desk at work. I even had an emergency container in my car that had snacks, not just survival food, but chips and granola bars!

Situation: When my kids were younger and I was a young mom and wife, getting everyone ready for the day, this is how a typical day would go for me. Get the kids up and ready for school, which entailed of cooking breakfast and preparing lunches. I'm eating breakfast as I'm preparing breakfast. Snacking on lunch food while I'm preparing lunches. Then as I drop them all off at their perspective locations of learning, and on my way to work, I would hit whichever drive through I was craving at the moment and consume whatever I fancied, the pleasure was in the exhale. It was a treat for me to eat without distraction or grubby little hands wanting my grown up food! Remember I

would also have food in my drawers at work. I was an administrative assistant (secretary/receptionist) at the time. So I would have community candy on my desk. People could always come to me for snacks! Oh and don't let there be a catering job that I was responsible for organizing, I would order everything that I wanted. And there were always left overs for me to consume as I finished out my day, or to take home, sometimes they didn't make it home. Then as the day ended, and it was time to pick the children up from school, I would stop at yet another drive thru and get what I desired. I would always get rid of the evidence before they got in the car asking a truck load of questions. Then I would get home and cook dinner, all the while nibbling and tasting as I went. After dinner was prepared, I would sit down to eat with my family. This behavior lasted for years. I believe ultimately that's what contributed to my gallstones.

At my restaurant, I'd find myself eating items that my customers would send back saying they didn't like something which was perfectly fine to me. I told my husband, at one point, that if I ate the way I thought about food, I would be easily 600 pounds! (Just so happens I think I'm kinda cute and my ego wouldn't allow me to get that size, so in this case vanity has worked to my advantage on some level.) We even had a refrigerator in our room so that if I didn't finish a meal that I was eating, I could put it in the fridge and wouldn't have to go downstairs to the kitchen to get my food when I wanted it again. Not to mention, by the time I got done eating, I was too lazy and stuffed to go all the way downstairs to put the food in the fridge. I still love eating in my bed while watching TV, NOT GOOD, and I still do it from time to time, but just don't make it a habit anymore.

Don't get me wrong, I still like food. It's not like I've given up food. I just know how to make better choices. When I go to the grocery store, if it's something that I'm wanting, I get a single portion of it, something that I can finish and is within my boundaries of a treat, and I eat it right then and there, never to enter my home. Instead of going to the fair and buying one of everything or at least tasting everything, I can choose what things I really want to try then share with someone I'm with. When I go to the movies, I don't have to order popcorn, and nachos, and a Slurpee, and ice-cream, and a hot dog, and anything else that seems interesting, I can simply just have a small popcorn and a drink while I'm watching the movie. Or I will make sure I eat a meal before I go to the movies, when I do that I typically don't want anything. If I sit down and eat a pizza, I don't have to consume a whole entire pizza by myself. However, if I feel like I want an entire pizza to myself, I will order a small one, and finish it off without guilt instead of fighting not to polish off a large one by myself.

There came a time that I realized that what I struggled with more than anything else, was the fact that I had no boundaries when my emotions were involved. The most dangerous emotion for me was anger. Even when I thought that there were boundaries to food, there really wasn't. I was addicted to food. The thing that I didn't realize was that when certain emotions displayed themselves, boundaries were non-existent. You may be in the same place with whatever emotion grips you most frequently and just don't realize it, because you never had an association with it. If you can simply pay attention to what emotion you are feeling when you are having a toxic relationship moment, then you will begin to be aware of what's happening and begin asking yourself questions. Why, what, when, how and where? If you're anything like me, it will take a while to acknowledge that food and or sugar is an addiction for you. What you're doing is unhealthy. You see, for me, I didn't have high blood pressure, my cholesterol was fine, I was not in jeopardy of diabetes, and when I went to the doctor, I got good reports; which made me think to myself that nothing is wrong with me, I'm just fat!

As I began to learn about proper eating, and to find out what just sugar and flour alone was doing to us, how to read the labels and see all of the ways that sugar has snuck into our food, it changed everything. It helped me to change my life. I want to help you change your life. What I've learned during my journey to step away from my addiction from food, is that with this step back, there's a sense of empowerment. I'm no longer bound by food. I have choices in life. I'm not a slave to the food or sugar anymore.

You too have the power to change your life. It's time for you to get this demon off your back. It doesn't have to be this way. I want to share with you my fights, my struggles. So you can see that there is also a light at the end of your tunnel. We no longer have to continue to kill ourselves through the diet that we eat. You can educate yourself just like I did. I began to read the labels of

EVERYTHING that I was going to put in my mouth. If it had any form of sugar, other than natural sugar, like say from real fruit, or real dairy, such as real cheese, milk or yogurt (plain) I just left it alone. I did this until I got a grip on my addiction.

My letter was a cry for help. It's a cry for help for me, and it's a cry for help for you. I know a lot of people feel that way, but they feel stuck, trapped, even imprisoned by food. They don't know how to verbalize what they are going through, and feel like no one understands, but let me tell you, I see you, I feel your pain and my prayer is for you to be healed through the words on these pages. I know it sounds cliché but honestly you are not alone. Food addiction is a disease of isolation and you don't have to be isolated any longer!

I'm here to help you change your current situation. I want to help educate you on what you're putting in your body, to show you how to begin to read labels and create boundaries in your life from food to anything else for that matter. You'd be surprised at how everything and everyone are really connected. A lot of us don't understand what we're reading when we're looking at the labels. I'm not talking about some kind of extreme diet where you become a vegan or vegetarian, unless of course you want to go that route, but just having an awareness of what you are putting in your body.

Our FB support group, Buxom Bodies in Motion is here to provide you resources. Different ways to get started, and the groups you can join like Whole30, Intermittent Fasting or the one that really helped me, FA, to really deal with your food addiction. This is not a one size fits all when it comes to this, but they can help you to understand what it really means to be and eat healthy, and of course this is a very mental process, so we need to get our minds right and healthy before we can make lifetime, lifestyle changes.

As part of our Facebook group, we can all work together to help one another through the process. I have videos that you can check out that show me in the grocery store showing how to read labels, to educate you what to look for.

What does processed food mean? What isn't processed food? We'll spend some time together learning how to prep meals. More than anything else, I want you to understand, what sugar really means for you. Forget for a minute, what your diabetic rating is, whether or not the doctor has, or hasn't diagnosed you as diabetic. You need to understand how toxic processed sugar is.

Being addicted to food, in general, is not a good way to live. It is, however, something that you can overcome. Like me, you may have just bought into the fact that you're overweight. Convinced yourself that there's no choice, that food's your friend and that this is the way life is. Or that it's okay because people accept you, or the doctor hasn't told you that you have problems.

I'm here to tell you there's a better way to live, that simply by taking small actions, to begin with, and joining us in a group of extremely supportive individuals. Then just committing yourself, first, to information; knowledge is power. When you begin to understand what you're putting into your body, you can then begin to develop better choices.

In closing, this brings us to not beating yourself up and loving yourself, just the way you are, where you are, by allowing yourself to choose in every area of your life! Ask yourself, "Do I feel like eating poison today?" I know it's a cold way to look at it, but if you are totally honest with yourself, you will see that this is a valid question, and even with that, you still have a choice. Is this something that I want to put into me? Many of us in our group have more than 100 pounds to lose, and if you're that woman, you're in the right place. (which by the way fat people are not the only ones addicted to food and sugar, with the others it just shows up differently for them) You don't have to worry anymore about being too embarrassed to participate; we have a safe space for you. A place where you can step out from that overwhelming toxic relationship that you've had with food, and you can make the bold step to say, "My dearest Food, I can never hate you, I can't live without you, but my Diabolically Delicious Toxic Relationship with you as I knew it……. is over."!

Respectfully,
Me